WEIGHT MAINTENANCE GUIDE

Holistic Therapies For Sustainable Weight Management

Achieve And Maintain A Healthy Weight Through A Holistic Approach To Weight Management And Innovative Therapies

DR. BRIDGET PROMISE

CHAPTER ONE 4

Introduction: 4

Knowing The Holistic Perspective 5

Examining The Relationship Between The
Mind And Body In Weight Loss 7

CHAPTER TWO 13

Including Exercise For A Balanced...............13

Strategies For Stress Reduction For 17

Good Sleep And Its Effect On.....................18

CHAPTER THREE 21

Mindful Eating: Fostering.......................21

Hormones And Their Effect On 24

Personalized Weight Loss Plans 28

CHAPTER FOUR 31

Comprehensive Strategies For 31

Creating Healthful Routines For Long-Term
Achievement 32

Social Support's Significance For...............34

Mind-Body Techniques For Reducing Stress
And Balancing Weight............................36

How to Design a Fun and Durable Exercise
Program 38

CHAPTER FIVE 40

Recognizing And Getting Past 40

Honoring Advancement: Contemplative
Evaluation Of The Weight Wellness Path 41

Keeping Things Balanced Outside 43

Summary 44

CHAPTER ONE

Introduction:

The idea of weight management has evolved beyond conventional paradigms in the ever-changing field of health and wellness, giving birth to a holistic approach that acknowledges the connection between the mind and body.

This all-encompassing viewpoint recognizes that maintaining a healthy weight requires more than simply tracking calories or following a tight diet. In this investigation, we look into the holistic approach to weight health, comprehending the importance of physical exercise for balanced well-being, the critical function of nutrition, and the complex mind-body relationship.

Knowing The Holistic Perspective On Weight Wellness:

The holistic approach to weight wellbeing focuses on a person's total health and happiness rather than just the outward look of their body.

It acknowledges that maintaining a healthy balance between the mind and body is just as important to weight control as just losing weight. This method takes into account several variables, such as stress management, lifestyle decisions, and emotional well-being, and it recognizes the critical roles these variables play in reaching and maintaining a healthy weight.

Adopting a holistic viewpoint entails realizing that problems related to weight are often complex. People struggle with their weight for a variety of reasons, such as psychological effects, environmental variables, and genetic predispositions. Recognizing the complexities of weight wellness allows people to approach their path with more compassion and understanding, emphasizing total health over giving in to social pressure or fast fixes.

Examining The Relationship Between The Mind And Body In Weight Loss

A key component of the holistic approach to weight health is the mind-body link. Our behaviors—including those about food and exercise—are greatly influenced by our ideas, feelings, and mental health.

For example, stress may lead to emotional eating, which can result in bad food choices and irregular eating habits. Long-term success in weight control requires an understanding of and attention to the underlying psychological problems that lead to weight difficulties.

A crucial element of the mind-body relationship is mindful eating. It entails developing a positive connection with food, being aware of hunger and fullness signals, and paying attention to the sensory experience of eating. Eating mindfully may assist people in making thoughtful decisions, enjoying the tastes of food, and creating a healthy connection with food.

Furthermore, it's critical to address the emotional factors that lead to overeating or harmful behaviors. People who possess emotional intelligence and coping strategies may effectively manage stress, anxiety, and other emotional obstacles without turning to unhealthful eating habits.

This all-encompassing strategy includes cultivating a mentality that promotes a healthy and long-lasting connection with food and body image in addition to behavior modification.

The Function of Diet in Maintaining a Sustainable Weight:

A key component of the holistic approach to weight health is nutrition. Adopting a nutritious and well-balanced eating plan that satisfies individual nutritional demands is prioritized above fad diets or severe limitations.

Entire, high-nutrient meals serve as the cornerstone for long-term weight management by giving the body the vital vitamins, minerals, and macronutrients it requires for optimum performance.

With this method, people are encouraged to see food as nourishment for their bodies rather than a cause for shame or limitation.

A well-rounded and fulfilling diet that supports an individual's overall health and weight objectives may be created by combining a range of fruits, vegetables, whole grains, lean meats, and healthy fats. A more thoughtful and pleasurable meal experience is also enhanced by mindful eating techniques like watching portion amounts and eating slowly.

The holistic approach to nutrition is significant because it takes individual preferences and variances into account. It acknowledges that there isn't a single, universally applicable remedy and exhorts individuals to discover a dietary regimen that suits their requirements and way of life.

This adaptability helps maintain weight healthiness over time by improving adherence to a healthy eating plan and cultivating a pleasant connection with food.

CHAPTER TWO

Including Exercise For A Balanced Well-Being:

A key element of the holistic approach to weight health is physical exercise. Apart from its function in burning calories and aiding in weight reduction, consistent exercise enhances general health and wellness. It supports the preservation of lean muscle mass and has a good effect on mood, energy levels, and cardiovascular health.

The holistic approach to physical exercise places a strong emphasis on the value of engaging in activities that people love. The idea is to partake in activities that make you happy and fulfilled, whether that means dancing, running, walking, swimming, or yoga. This improves the sustainability of exercise and fosters a favorable attitude toward physical activity.

It is also stressed that adding strength training to the exercise regimen is important since it helps to retain muscle mass, increase metabolism, and promote functional fitness. To enhance general health and fitness, the holistic approach recommends a well-rounded regimen of cardiovascular, strength, and flexibility training.

Additionally, exercise is acknowledged as a very effective stress-reduction strategy. Frequent exercise has been shown to lower stress hormones, lessen depressive and anxious symptoms, and enhance mental toughness in general.

People may improve their capacity to handle life's obstacles by addressing the mind-body link via physical exercise, which helps to promote a more holistic and well-rounded approach to weight well-being.

In summary, the holistic approach to weight well-being highlights the connection between the mind and body and signifies a paradigm change in our knowledge of health. People may control their weight in a more compassionate and long-lasting way by acknowledging the complexity of weight issues and taking care of the mind-body link.

In this journey, nutrition is crucial since it promotes a healthy, well-balanced diet that supports general health. Incorporating physical exercise also serves as a way to improve overall wellness by supporting resilience on the mental and emotional levels in addition to weight management. A good connection with one's body may be cultivated, leading to long-term health and happiness, by adopting a holistic approach to weight wellness.

Strategies For Stress Reduction For A Healthy Weight

Achieving the objective of maintaining a healthy weight often requires making a variety of lifestyle and dietary decisions. Stress management is an important but sometimes disregarded component. The complicated link between stress and weight arises from the fact that, depending on an individual's response to stress, stress may cause both weight increase and reduction. We'll talk about stress-reduction strategies in this session that support reaching and maintaining a healthy weight.

Good Sleep And Its Effect On Wellness And Weight

It is impossible to overestimate the importance of getting enough good sleep to attain general well-being, which includes keeping a healthy weight. Sleep is essential for maintaining hormone balance, metabolism, and energy balance. These vital processes may be upset by persistently getting little or poor-quality sleep, which might result in problems with weight.

Hormones like ghrelin and leptin that regulate appetite and hunger may be impacted by sleep loss. Lack of sleep causes a rise in ghrelin, often known as the hunger hormone, which tells the body to consume more. However, there is a leptin drop, the hormone that signals fullness, which increases the risk of overheating. An environment that is favorable to weight growth is produced by this hormonal imbalance.

Moreover, a lack of sleep might affect the body's capacity to control blood sugar levels, raising the possibility of developing insulin resistance. Reduced insulin sensitivity may make it difficult for the body to properly regulate glucose, which can eventually lead to weight gain and the emergence of diseases like type 2 diabetes.

Developing a sleep-friendly atmosphere and forming good sleep habits should be people's top priorities if they want to increase the quality of their sleep.

CHAPTER THREE

Mindful Eating: Fostering Consciousness With Each Bite

Eating mindfully is a technique that helps people focus on the here and now while they are eating. Many individuals in our fast-paced environment eat while on the move or while occupied with other tasks, which may result in mindless eating and overindulgence.

The goal of mindful eating is to increase awareness of the whole eating process, from choosing foods to consuming them.

People who practice mindfulness during meals might become more aware of their bodies' signals of hunger and fullness. Choosing what, when, and how much to consume becomes easier with this increased knowledge.

Studies have shown that engaging in mindful eating practices may result in better eating habits, less emotional eating, and enhanced control over weight.

Savoring every mouthful and taking in the tastes, textures, and scents of the meal is a key component of mindful eating. This methodical approach to eating may increase pleasure with fewer servings and create a stronger bond with the culinary experience.

Furthermore, mindful eating promotes a more intuitive approach to eating by teaching people to listen to their bodies' signals of hunger and fullness.

By learning to accept their body's natural signals, people may develop a better connection with food instead of depending on external cues or restrictive diets.

Hormones And Their Effect On Body Composition

Hormones are essential for controlling several physiological functions, such as body composition and metabolism. Stress, both acute and chronic, may upset these hormones' delicate balance and may be a factor in weight-related problems.

Cortisol, also known as the stress hormone, is one important hormone impacted by stress. Cortisol levels increase in reaction to perceived danger, priming the body for the "fight or flight" response. Although in times of acute stress, this reaction is necessary for survival, long-term stress may result in persistently high cortisol levels, which can contribute to weight gain.

Elevated cortisol levels can increase hunger, especially for meals heavy in fat and sugar. This may result in overindulging, particularly under pressure. Furthermore, cortisol encourages fat accumulation, especially in the vicinity of the abdomen. An elevated risk of cardiovascular illnesses and other health problems is linked to this visceral fat.

Prolonged stress may also influence other hormones, such as thyroid and insulin, which can further impair the body's capacity to control weight. Elevated blood sugar and fat accumulation may result from insulin resistance, which is often linked to stress.

It is essential to include stress-reduction techniques in everyday living to manage stress and its hormonal effects.

These might include doing deep breathing exercises, practicing mindfulness meditation, getting regular exercise, and partaking in enjoyable and soothing hobbies.

People may promote a healthy body composition and favorably impact hormone balance by treating the underlying cause of stress.

To sum up, controlling stress is essential to reaching and keeping a healthy weight. A comprehensive approach to weight health includes getting enough sleep, practicing mindful eating, and being aware of how hormones affect body composition. Through the integration of stress management strategies into their everyday lives, people may establish a basis for sustained health and overall well-being.

Personalized Weight Loss Plans And Functional Medicine

The approach to weight management has changed beyond the traditional one-size-fits-all techniques in the quest for optimum health and well-being. The advent of functional medicine has resulted in a paradigm change in our comprehension and management of weight-related concerns.

To build specific weight management strategies, this holistic approach takes into account not only the physical elements of weight but also individual examinations and the integration of conventional and alternative treatments.

Combining Conventional and complementary therapies

Because every individual is different and may react differently to different treatments, functional medicine recognizes this and integrates standard medical procedures with alternative therapies. This method of weight management recognizes that individual differences exist in the causes that lead to weight increase or difficulties in decreasing weight.

Complementing traditional treatments like diet programs and exercise regimens are complementary therapies like herbal medicine, acupuncture, and mindfulness training. Practitioners hope to treat the underlying causes of weight-related problems by combining several modalities while keeping in mind the interdependence of the body's systems.

CHAPTER FOUR

Comprehensive Strategies For Emotional Eating

The understanding of the emotional factors connected to eating patterns is a key component of functional medicine's approach to weight control. Functional medicine offers holistic methods to treat the underlying reasons for emotional eating as opposed to just calorie tracking and restricted diets.

Personalized weight control regimens use therapeutic approaches including mindfulness exercises and cognitive-behavioral therapy. These methods enable people to make thoughtful decisions and break away from bad eating habits by giving them a better knowledge of their connection with food.

Creating Healthful Routines For Long-Term Achievement

The focus on creating long-lasting, healthful behaviors is one of the main tenets of functional medicine. In contrast to fast fixes, which often lead to short-term weight reduction, functional medicine seeks to establish lifelong lifestyle modifications in patients.

Personalized weight-management programs put a lot of emphasis on setting attainable objectives that are specific to each person's requirements and situation. This might include introducing fun physical activities, making progressive dietary adjustments, and taking care of any underlying medical conditions that could be causing weight problems. Functional medicine encourages long-lasting changes that transcend the scale by placing a higher priority on long-term well-being than on immediate outcomes.

Social Support's Significance For Weight Wellness

Understanding that maintaining good health is a team effort, functional medicine emphasizes the role that social support plays in weight well-being. Whether it be via local meet-ups, online forums, or group therapy, interacting with a supportive community may be very important for someone trying to control their weight.

Social support creates a supportive atmosphere for those pursuing weight-related objectives by offering a feeling of connection, empathy, and encouragement. It may serve as a forum for experience sharing and learning from others who have gone through similar problems, as well as a source of encouragement during trying times.

To sum up, functional medicine has ushered in a new era of customized weight-management regimens that surpass traditional methods. Functional medicine provides a thorough and all-encompassing framework for people seeking long-term weight wellness by emphasizing the value of social support, addressing the emotional aspects of eating, integrating conventional and alternative therapies, and encouraging healthy habits. This method takes into account both the physical components of weight and the complex interactions between many variables that affect a person's overall well-being.

Mind-Body Techniques For Reducing Stress And Balancing Weight

The achievement of general well-being is contingent upon the integration of the mind and body. Mind-body techniques, including yoga and meditation, provide a potent way to manage stress and maintain a healthy weight. These techniques emphasize coordinating breath awareness with physical motions to foster mental clarity and calm. In addition to reducing stress, practicing mindfulness may have a good effect on eating habits by encouraging a thoughtful attitude to food intake.

Yoga offers a variety of alternatives ideal for different levels of fitness due to its varying styles and intensities. Incorporating regulated breathing, soft postures, and meditation may help lower stress levels and increase awareness of your body's signals. By encouraging healthy choices in food and exercise, this mindful connection lays the groundwork for long-term weight control.

How to Design a Fun and Durable Exercise Program

It's important to keep workout regimens sustainable. The path to weight well-being has to be pleasurable, flexible, and simple to integrate into daily existence. While intense exercise regimens and fad diets may provide short-term improvements, they often lack the durability needed for long-term weight control.

A good exercise regimen should include things that you like and feel fulfilled with. This might include everything from more formal gym routines to dancing, hiking, or cycling.

Finding something that meshes well with one's hobbies and daily routine is crucial. By lowering stress and producing endorphins, a long-term workout regimen helps control weight and improve mental health in general.

CHAPTER FIVE

Recognizing And Getting Past Weight Management Plateaus

It might be demoralizing to have weight control plateaus, which are typical. It is essential to understand the causes of plateaus to overcome them. A regular exercise regimen or diet plan might cause the body to adjust, which can temporarily stop weight loss or muscle building.

The remedy to plateaus is variety. One way to shock the body back into responsiveness is to introduce new activities, tweak eating habits, or increase the intensity of workouts. Additionally, it's essential to maintain a well-balanced diet and pay attention to the nutritional value of meals. Consulting with fitness experts or dietitians might provide tailored approaches to break through obstacles and keep moving forward with your weight-wellness goal.

Honoring Advancement: Contemplative Evaluation Of The Weight Wellness Path

Setting objectives is not as crucial as recognizing accomplishments in the quest for weight health. People who practice mindful reflection can recognize and value all of their accomplishments, no matter how great or little. This encouragement not only increases motivation but also improves the road toward health as a whole.

For development to be maintained, reasonable objectives must be set and broken down into achievable increments. Maintaining a positive outlook and recognizing the little victories along the way strengthens the will to achieve long-term weight health. Every success, whether it's losing a few pounds, hitting a workout goal, or making better food choices, should be acknowledged.

Keeping Things Balanced Outside Of The Scale

There's more to managing weight than just the numbers on the scale. It entails developing a well-rounded lifestyle that takes mental, emotional, and physical health into account. Although weight is a quantifiable measure, focusing too much on it might result in an imbalanced and sometimes harmful attitude toward well-being.

Embracing balance is putting mental health first, cultivating wholesome relationships, and using mindfulness techniques to reduce stress. Including pleasant physical activities in everyday life improves general health and well-being, regardless of their effect on weight. The objective is to sustain a whole feeling of health and vigor rather than merely reaching a certain weight.

Summary

To sum up, achieving lifetime weight health is a dynamic and comprehensive undertaking. This all-encompassing approach includes mind-body techniques for stress reduction, the development of long-lasting exercise regimens, the recognition and acceptance of plateaus, the celebration of accomplishments, and the maintenance of balance outside of physical boundaries.

By understanding how mental and physical health interact, people may develop a fulfilling and sustainable lifestyle that supports healthy weight management. In addition to losing weight, the goal is to create a healthy, balanced connection between the body and mind, which will set the stage for a lifetime of holistic health and well-being.